50 Recipes for GERD Patients

Keep GERD on A Low with This Cookbook

By

Heston Brown

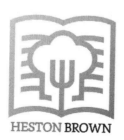

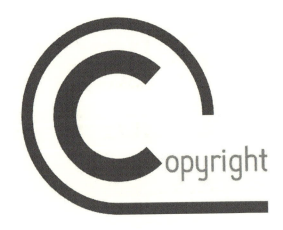

Copyright 2019 Heston Brown

All rights reserved. No part of this Book should be reproduced by any means including but not limited to: digital or mechanical copies, printed copies, scanning or photocopying unless approval is given by the Owner of the Book.

Any suggestions, guidelines or ideas in the Book are purely informative and the Author assumes no responsibility for any burden, loss, or damage caused by a misunderstanding of the information contained therein. The Reader assumes any and all risk when following information contained in the Book.

Thank you so much for buying my book! I want to give you a special gift!

Receive a special gift as a thank you for buying my book. Now you will be able to benefit from free and discounted book offers that are sent directly to your inbox every week.

To subscribe simply fill in the box below with your details and start reaping the rewards! A new deal will arrive every day and reminders will be sent so you never miss out. Fill in the box below to subscribe and get started!

https://heston-brown.getresponsepages.com

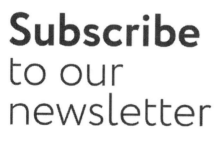

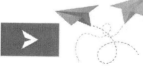

Table of Contents

Chapter I - Casseroles 8

Recipe 1: Shredded Beef Casserole 9

Recipe 2: Italian Pork Casserole.. 11

Recipe 3: Taco Casserole 13

Recipe 4: GERD Friendly Chicken and Rice...................... 15

Recipe 5: Baked Chicken Salad 17

Recipe 6: Deliciously Lite Tuna Casserole......................... 19

Recipe 7: Burn Free Tetrazzini 21

Recipe 8: Flare Free Cordon Blue 23

Recipe 9: Teriyaki Shrimp and Noodles 25

Recipe 10: Honey Biscuits, Broccoli and Ham 27

Chapter II - Lunch 29

Recipe 1: Ham Wraps 30

Recipe 2: Reflux Free Pot Pie 33

Recipe 3: Chicken Pitas 35

Recipe 4: Homemade Chicken Drummies 37

Recipe 5: Asian Chicken Tenders a GERD Friendly Cool Honey Mustard Dipping Sauce 39

Recipe 6: Easy Chicken Wraps 42

Recipe 7: Lunchtime Chicken Kabobs 44

Recipe 8: Cubed Steak Sandwiches 46

Recipe 9: Mushroom Fettuccine 48

Recipe 10: Sweet and Sour Chicken Roll Ups 50

Chapter III - Dinner 52

Recipe 1: Turkey with Sweet Potato Wedges 53

Recipe 2: Faux Fried Chicken 55

Recipe 3: Turkey and Tofu Green Beans 57

Recipe 4: Burn Free Shrimp Pasta 59

Recipe 5: White Lasagna 61

Recipe 6: Thyme Ribs 63

Recipe 7: Piece O'Beef Kabobs 65

Recipe 8: Honey Chicken 67

Recipe 9: Spinach and Shrimp Parmesan Linguine 70

Recipe 10: GERD Stroganoff 72

Chapter IV - Stews 75

Recipe 1: Chickpea and Spinach Stew 76

Recipe 2: Pork and Sweet Potato Stew 78

Recipe 3: Beef and Broccoli Stew Version 2 81

Recipe 4: Beef and Broccoli Stew 83

Recipe 5: Cornmeal Veggie Stew 85

Recipe 6: Chicken and Herbed Biscuits 87

Recipe 7: Herbed Chicken Stew 89

Recipe 8: Bok Choy Stew 91

Recipe 9: Shrimp and Corn Stew 93

Recipe 10: Ham and Broccoli Stew 95

Chapter V - Snacks and Desserts 97

Recipe 1: GERD Approved Banana Bread 98

Recipe 2: Chicken Pot Pie Muffins 100

Recipe 3: Vanilla Ice Cream Strawberry Cake 102

Recipe 4: Apple Crumble Muffins 104

Recipe 5: Italian Half's 106

Recipe 6: Orange Bites 108

Recipe 7: Baked Shrimp Won Tons 110

Recipe 8: Baked Fritters 112

Recipe 9: Baked Vegetarian Spring Rolls 114

Recipe 10: Black Cherry Yogurt Pops 116

Recipe 11: Tuna Salad Celery Dips 118

About the Author 120

Author's Afterthoughts 122

Chapter I - Casseroles

Recipe 1: Shredded Beef Casserole

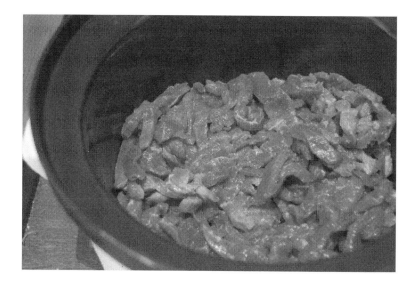

London broil's are high in vitamin c! 1 serving

List of Ingredients:

- 1 medium to large London broil
- 1 head of cauliflower
- 4 large basil leaves chopped
- ½ Tbsp. brown sugar
- ¼ cup apple cider vinegar
- ¼ cup olive oil
- 2 cup low sodium, low fat chicken broth
- 1 tsp. black pepper

xxxxxxxxxxxxxxxxxxxxxxxxxxxxxxxxxxx

Instructions:

Marinate London broil overnight in olive oil, apple cider vinegar, brown sugar and basil. Using a food processor pulse in short rapid burst until cauliflower is in rice size pieces. In crockpot pour the marinade and the London broil, cook for 5 ½ hours then shred. Add cauliflower rice, broth, and pepper, mix together and let cook another 30 minutes. Serve.

Recipe 2: Italian Pork Casserole

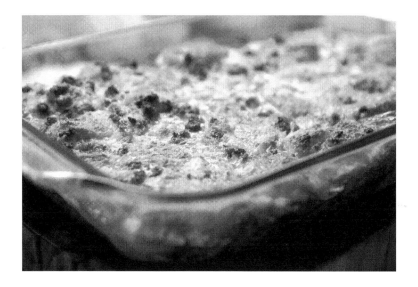

Works with beef too! Makes 4

List of Ingredients:

- 3-4 cups Pork stew pieces
- 1 cup brown rice
- 1 Tbsp. Italian seasoning
- ¼ cup diced celery
- 2 cups low sodium beef broth

xxxxxxxxxxxxxxxxxxxxxxxxxxxxxxxxxxxxxx

Instructions:

Preheat oven to 350 and prepare a 9x11 casserole dish

Brown the pork pieces and let sit on a paper towel 5-8 minutes; meanwhile, pour uncooked rice into dish, top with seasonings and celery, pour in broth and stir well. Add pork pieces and cook, uncovered 45-50 minutes

Recipe 3: Taco Casserole

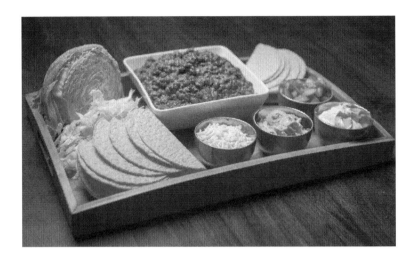

Try various seasonings and discover your favorite! Makes 1 9x11 casserole, approx. 10-12 servings

List of Ingredients:

- 1 bag low sodium, low fat tortilla chips, crushed
- 1-pound lean ground beef, browned and drained
- 1 cup cheddar cheese or Mexican blend
- 1/3 cup diced scallions
- 2/3 cup black beans, washed and dried
- Salt-Free Mexican seasoning

xxxxxxxxxxxxxxxxxxxxxxxxxxxxxxxxxxxxxx

Instructions:

Preheat oven to 425 and prepare 9x11 casserole dish

In a bowl, mix all of the ingredients together; pour into dish and bake 10-12 minutes.

Recipe 4: GERD Friendly Chicken and Rice

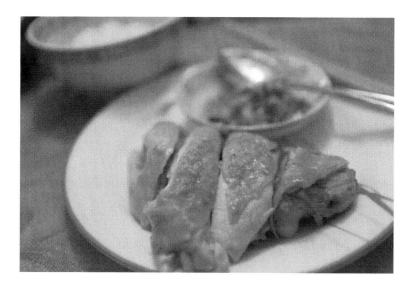

As usual, opt for low-fat varieties of ingredients! Makes 2 servings

List of Ingredients:

- 2 boneless, skinless chicken breast
- 3/4 cup rice
- 1/3 cup fat free cream of mushroom condensed soup
- 1/3 tsp. black pepper
- 1/3 Tbsp. diced rosemary
- 2 cups water

xxxxxxxxxxxxxxxxxxxxxxxxxxxxxxxxxxxxx

Instructions:

Preheat oven to 350 and prepare a 9x9 casserole dish

In a 9x9 casserole dish pour in rice, place chicken on top, mix mushroom soup, rosemary, and pepper into water and pour into dish. Cook, covered, thirty minutes, uncover, and cook 15 more minutes.

Recipe 5: Baked Chicken Salad

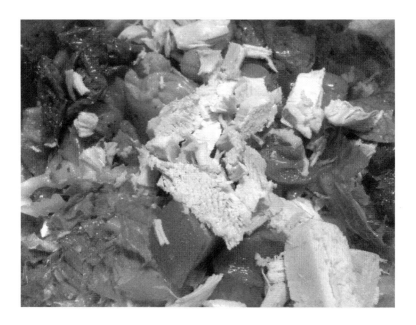

Great light casserole for warm nights! Makes 10-12 nuggets

List of Ingredients:

- 1 cup diced boneless skinless chicken breast or thighs, browned
- 1 head chopped bok choy
- 2 cups broccoli slaw
- 2 cup mushrooms
- 1/6 tsp. cinnamon
- 3 cups low sodium, low fat chicken broth
- 1 tsp. Worchester sauce

xxxxxxxxxxxxxxxxxxxxxxxxxxxxxxxxxxxx

Instructions:

Prepare crockpot and brown chicken pieces

Place all ingredients and liquids into chamber; cook on high 45 minutes to 1 hour

Recipe 6: Deliciously Lite Tuna Casserole

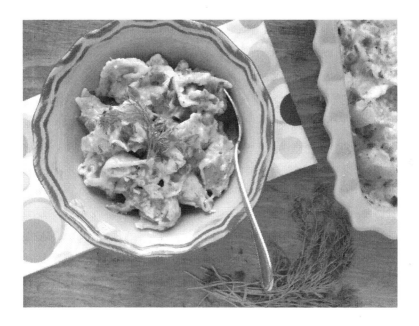

Be sure to get tuna packed in water! Makes 4 servings

List of Ingredients:

- 1 can or pack tuna
- 6-8 oz. noodles (little shells, rigatoni, etc.)
- 1/3 cup diced celery
- 1 tsp. chives
- 1/3 cup mayonnaise
- 1/3 cup cream of celery or mushroom condensed soup
- 1/3 cup water
- ½ cup plain breadcrumbs
- Parmesan cheese

xxxxxxxxxxxxxxxxxxxxxxxxxxxxxxxxxxxx

Instructions:

Preheat oven to 400 and prepare a 9x9 casserole dish

Let noodles boil 8 minutes; meanwhile, mix together tuna, celery, chives, mayo, and condensed soup. Drain noodles, do not rinse, and stir into tuna/mayo mix; pour into dish top with breadcrumbs and cheese. Cook 30-35 minutes

Recipe 7: Burn Free Tetrazzini

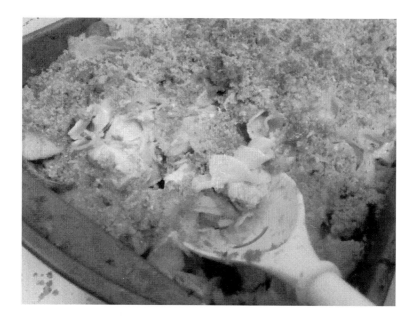

Chicken, turkey, pork, or seafood works great in this recipe!

Makes 4-6 servings

List of Ingredients:

- 1 cup shredded beef
- 1 Tbsp. butter
- 1 cup diced mushrooms
- 1 Tbsp. brown sugar
- 1 Tbsp. all-purpose flour
- 1 dash Worchester sauce
- 1 cup chicken broth
- 1/3 cup Marsala
- Mashed potatoes or wide egg noodles

xxxxxxxxxxxxxxxxxxxxxxxxxxxxxxxxxxx

Instructions:

Preheat oven to 350 and prepare a 9x9 casserole dish

In a large pot melt butter into mushrooms, and brown sugar; add flour, Worchester sauce, chicken broth, and marsala; bring to a boil reduce add beef; fill the bottom of dish with cooked mashed potatoes or noodles and top with beef mix. Cook 30 minutes

Recipe 8: Flare Free Cordon Blue

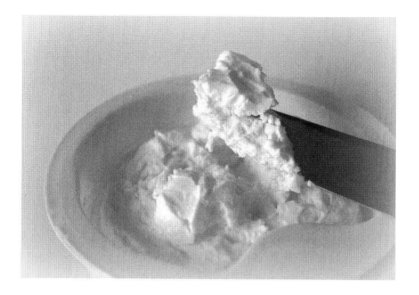

Serve with a salad or crusty bread! Makes 2 servings

List of Ingredients:

- 1 cup worth diced chicken
- 1 cup of diced ham
- 4 oz. low fat cream cheese
- 1/3 stick butter
- pepper
- ½ tsp. blue monde seasoning (if doesn't cause flaring, if it does it can be omitted)
- ½ Tbsp. thyme or oregano or rosemary

xxxxxxxxxxxxxxxxxxxxxxxxxxxxxxxxxx

Instructions:

Preheat oven to 350 and prepare a 9x11 casserole dish

In pot over med. High melt butter and cream cheese, add spices and seasonings, finally add proteins, stir, and cook 7-10 minutes. Pour into casserole dish and bake 40-45 minutes.

Recipe 9: Teriyaki Shrimp and Noodles

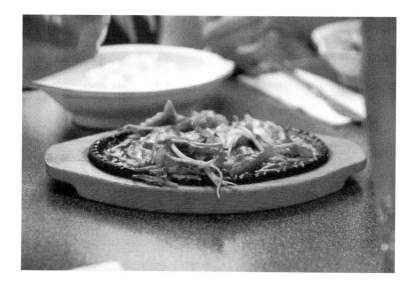

Frozen vegetables work just as good as canned! Makes 8-10 servings

List of Ingredients:

- ½ pound shrimp, cleaned, deveined, and de-tailed
- 1 can chow mein vegetables
- 1 cup rice
- 2 cups water
- 2 Tbsp. honey
- 3 Tbsp. melted butter
- ½ Tbsp. Worchester sauce or soy sauce

xxxxxxxxxxxxxxxxxxxxxxxxxxxxxxxxxxxx

Instructions:

Preheat oven to 350 and prepare a 9x11 casserole dish

In plastic bag pour honey, melted butter, sauce of choice, and prepared shrimp and let sit in refrigerator anywhere from 30 minutes to 2 hours. In casserole dish mix together rice, water vegetables, and marinated shrimp; cook, uncovered 30-35 minutes

Recipe 10: Honey Biscuits, Broccoli and Ham

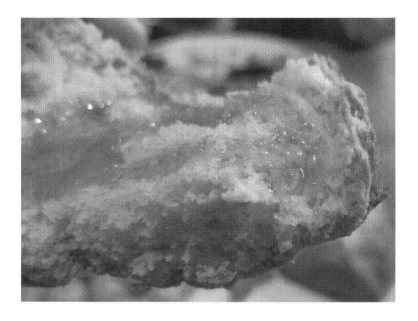

A savory meal for all to enjoy! Makes 8-10 servings

List of Ingredients:

- 1 large can frozen biscuits
- 1 cup chopped broccoli
- 1 cup diced ham
- 1/3 cup honey
- 1 Tbsp. butter, melted
- Italian seasoning (optional)

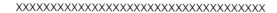

Instructions:

Preheat oven to 425 and prepare 9x11 casserole dish

Split in half and lay face up in casserole dish; top with broccoli and ham, spreading out evenly.

Mix honey, melted butter, and any spices, herbs, or seasonings in small bowl and cook 12-14 minutes

Chapter II - Lunch

Recipe 1: Ham Wraps

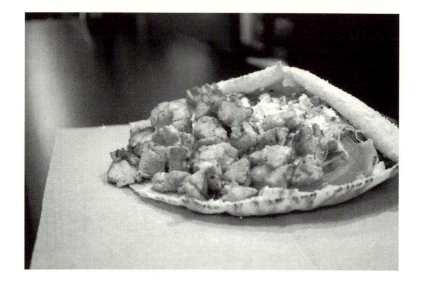

For an extra kick add honey and a dash of black pepper to the vinaigrette! Makes 2 servings

List of Ingredients:

- 2 low salt, low fat wraps
- 2/3 cup low sodium diced ham
- ½ cup bok choy, kale, or spinach
- 1/3 cup diced black olives
- Parmesan cheese (optional)
- ½ cup Home-made Vinaigrette dressing (see below for recipe)

Home-Made Vinaigrette:

- Approx. 1 cup
- ½ cup olive oil
- 1 tsp. rosemary
- 1/3 cup red wine vinegar
- 1/8 tsp. cloves
- ½ tsp. garlic
- ½ tsp. red pepper flakes

xxxxxxxxxxxxxxxxxxxxxxxxxxxxxxxxxxxx

Instructions:

In large mixing bowl stir together diced ham, greens, eggplant, and 1/3 cup of home-made dressing. Vinaigrette will keep for 3-5 days in an airtight container in the refrigerator; always s hake well before serving. Fill Wraps with ham mixture and cheese

Recipe 2: Reflux Free Pot Pie

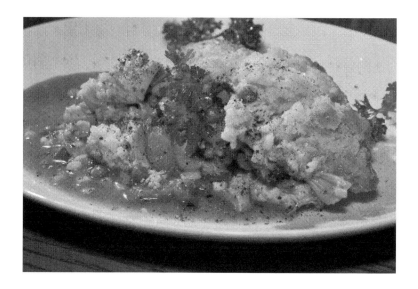

As with all recipes, use fat free and low sodium ingredients; makes 1 pie approx. 7-8 servings

List of Ingredients:

- 1 cup finely diced or shredded chicken
- ½ cup chicken broth
- 1/3 cup fat free cream of chicken condensed soup
- 1 drained can mixed vegetables
- 1 package phyllo dough
- 1 egg white
- Dash of cinnamon (optional)

xxxxxxxxxxxxxxxxxxxxxxxxxxxxxxxxxx

Instructions:

Preheat oven to 325 and prepare a 9x9 casserole dish

Lay out dough 3-5 minutes before working with, cut dough sheets to size to cover bottom and sides of dish. Lay a few sheets of phyllo dough and set aside; mix together broth and condensed soup, veggies, and chicken. Cover with dough, with pastry brush paint with egg white and cinnamon, and bake uncovered for 28-32 minutes

Recipe 3: Chicken Pitas

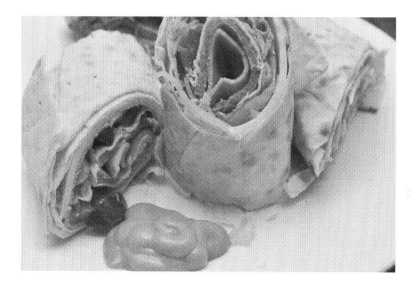

Also great on flatbread, in a wrap, or as a dip! Makes 3-4 sandwich's

List of Ingredients:

- 3-4 pita shells
- 1 can of chicken, or, 1 cup finely diced chicken breast or thigh, or, 1 cup shredded chicken
- 1 can low sodium, chickpeas washed and dried
- 1 dash lemon juice
- 1 tsp. garlic powder and parsley
- 1 tsp. red pepper flakes
- ½ tsp. orange peel

xxxxxxxxxxxxxxxxxxxxxxxxxxxxxxxxxxxx

Instructions:

Mix chickpeas, lemon juice, garlic powder and parsley, red pepper flakes, and orange peel together and puree; add chicken to mix and stir, spoon inside pitas

Recipe 4: Homemade Chicken Drummies

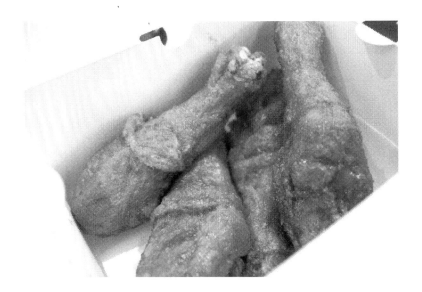

Don't worry; the name is deceiving you won't have to start raising chickens! Makes 8 drummies, 2-3 servings

List of Ingredients:

- 8 drummies, cleaned and dried
- ½ cup molasses
- 1/3 cup honey
- ¼ cup apple cider vinegar
- 1 Tbsp. olive oil
- 1 Tbsp. brown sugar
- ½ Tbsp. diced basil

xxxxxxxxxxxxxxxxxxxxxxxxxxxxxxxxxxx

Instructions:

Preheat oven to 350 and prepare baking tray

In pot over med.- high heat mix together molasses, honey, apple cider vinegar, olive oil, brown sugar, and basil; bring to boil, reduce heat, and simmer 28-30 minutes stirring occasionally. Brush onto drummies and cook 35-45 minutes.

Recipe 5: Asian Chicken Tenders a GERD Friendly Cool Honey Mustard Dipping Sauce

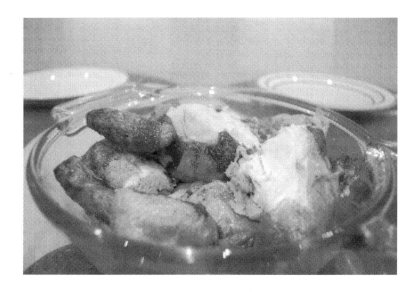

When you crave something "different" these hit the spot!

Makes 8

List of Ingredients:

- 8 chicken tenders
- 1/3 cup honey
- 1 tsp. low sodium soy sauce
- 1/3 Tbsp. pineapple juice
- 1/3 Tbsp. brown sugar
- 1 dash red pepper flakes (optional)
- Sesame seeds

Sauce

- 1/3 cup plain mustard
- 1 ½ honey
- 1/3 Tbsp. olive oil
- 1 tsp. soy sauce
- 1 Tbsp. diced basil and rosemary

xxxxxxxxxxxxxxxxxxxxxxxxxxxxxxxxxxxx

Instructions:

Preheat oven to 375 and prepare a baking tray

In plastic bag place all liquids, honey, red pepper flakes (if using), chicken tenders and let sit 4-6 hours. Lie on tray, sprinkle with sesame seeds and bake 30 minutes. For the sauce, mix all ingredients together and transfer to dipping bowls. Make the dipping sauce ahead and keep in air tight containers in the refrigerator.

Recipe 6: Easy Chicken Wraps

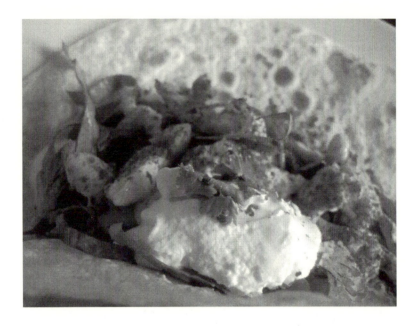

Also works great with canned meats such as shrimp and ham!

Makes 4 wraps

List of Ingredients:

- Leftover shredded chicken or ½ can chicken pieces
- 1/3 head romaine lettuce or kale
- 1/3 cup carrot matchsticks
- ½ Tbsp. honey
- 1/3 Tbsp. mustard
- 1 dash red pepper flakes
- 1 tsp. diced basil

xxxxxxxxxxxxxxxxxxxxxxxxxxxxxxxxxxxx

Instructions:

Lay out wraps on flat surface. In small bowl mix together honey, mustard, apple cider vinegar, red pepper flakes, and basil; in another bowl place chicken and carrot matchsticks. Mix the sauce into the carrot mix, lay lettuce/kale pieces on wraps and spoon 2 heaping spoonful's onto it.

Recipe 7: Lunchtime Chicken Kabobs

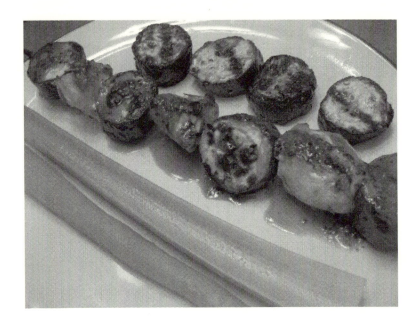

Light and healthy! Makes 4

List of Ingredients:

- 1 chicken breast cut into 2x3 chunks
- 1 eggplant cut into 2x3 pieces
- 1 zucchini cut into thin rounds
- 1 Tbsp. brown sugar
- ¼ cup olive oil
- 1 Tbsp. diced basil or rosemary

xxxxxxxxxxxxxxxxxxxxxxxxxxxxxxxxxxxxx

Instructions:

Turn on broiler, prepare ingredients, and soak 4 skewers

In a bowl mix together brown sugar, olive oil, and spices; place pieces on skewers, put under broiler 4-6 minutes

Recipe 8: Cubed Steak Sandwiches

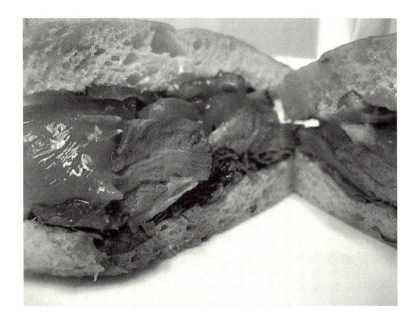

Great for a quick afternoon pick-me-up! Makes 2 sandwiches

List of Ingredients:

- 2 pieces of cubed steak
- 2 sandwich buns
- ½ Tbsp. butter
- 1/3 Tbsp. olive oil
- ½ cup flour
- 1/3 Tbsp. diced parsley, oregano, rosemary

xxxxxxxxxxxxxxxxxxxxxxxxxxxxxxxxxxxxxx

Instructions:

In bowl mix together flour and herbs and coated meat; make a mix of melted butter and olive oil in skillet and cook steaks 3-4 minutes on each side. Let sit on a paper towel 1-2 minutes before placing on bun and serving

Recipe 9: Mushroom Fettuccine

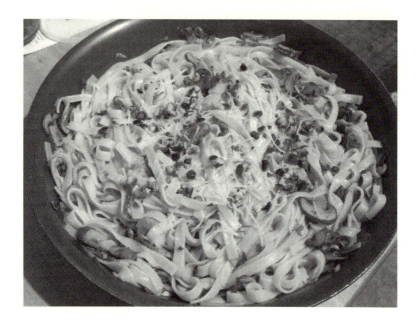

An easy crockpot meal good for unexpected guests! Makes 4-6 servings

List of Ingredients:

- 1 cup chopped button or shitake mushrooms
- 1 diced boneless, skinless chicken breast or 2 thighs, browned
- 1/3 cup cornmeal
- 1/3 Tbsp. butter
- ½ tub low fat sour cream
- 1 packet low sodium chicken broth
- ½ Tbsp. diced thyme or oregano
- ½ - 2/3 8 oz. box of fettuccine

xxxxxxxxxxxxxxxxxxxxxxxxxxxxxxxxxxxx

Instructions:

Before cooking lightly coat chicken in cornmeal and brown; let rest on paper towel during set up. In crockpot put in sour cream, butter, chicken broth, and stir well; mix in chicken pieces, mushrooms, and herbs. Let cook on high 30 minutes, add in fettuccine and continue cooking on high 30 minutes more.

Recipe 10: Sweet and Sour Chicken Roll Ups

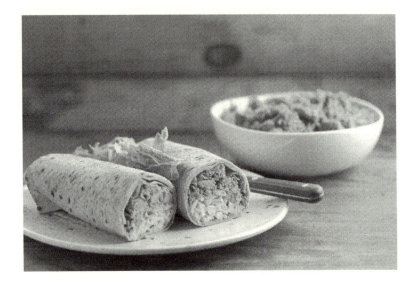

The tiny amount of pineapple juice used should be ok but I listed some alternatives just in case! Makes 8 roll ups

List of Ingredients:

- ½ Tbsp. pineapple juice or apple cider vinegar
- ½ Tbsp. soy sauce or Worchester sauce or vanilla extract
- 2 cups shredded chicken, or, 2 chicken breasts pound down to 1 inch and cut into thin strips
- 4 10-inch flour tortilla rolls
- 1 package shredded cheddar cheese
- Olive oil

xxxxxxxxxxxxxxxxxxxxxxxxxxxxxxxxxxxxx

Instructions:

Preheat oven to 325 and prepare a baking sheet

Marinade chicken in 2 liquids 3-4 hours, lay tortillas out and sprinkle each with cheese, fill one side with chicken and roll.

With a brush coat the open edge and the rest of the rolled tortilla with oil and lay edge side down. Bake 27-30 minutes, let cool for ten minutes and cut in half

Chapter III - Dinner

Recipe 1: Turkey with Sweet Potato Wedges

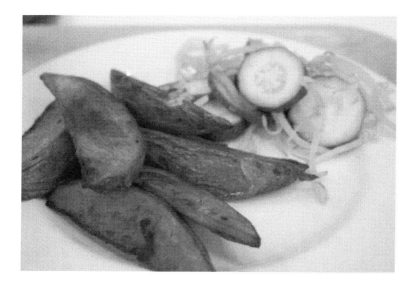

Turkey is a great lean protein! Makes 2 servings

List of Ingredients:

- 4 slices of French bread roll
- 2 turkey fillet
- Olive oil for sprinkling
- 1 tsp. brown sugar
- 1 tsp. diced thyme leaves
- 1/3 tsp. onion powder
- ½ tsp. garlic powder
- 1 large sweet potato cut into wedges (4 oz.)

xxxxxxxxxxxxxxxxxxxxxxxxxxxxxxxxx

Instructions:

Preheat oven to 350, prepare skillet, and a baking sheet

Mix together brown sugar, thyme, onion powder, and garlic powder; cut sweet potatoes into wedges and sprinkle with seasoning. Spread on tray and bake 45 minutes; meanwhile, cook fillets in skillet. If desired, toast buns under broiler with smear of butter on each slice

Recipe 2: Faux Fried Chicken

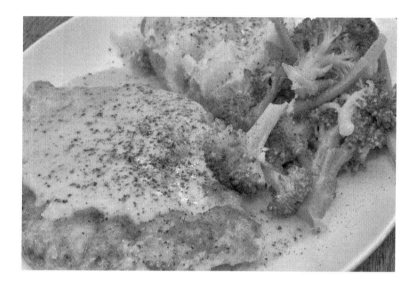

Also heart healthy and lower in cholesterol! Serves 2

List of Ingredients:

- 2 skinless, boneless chicken breasts
- 1/3 cup olive oil
- ½ Tbsp. apple cider vinegar *
- 2 Tbsp. brown sugar
- ½ cup buttermilk cornmeal

xxxxxxxxxxxxxxxxxxxxxxxxxxxxxxxxxxx

Instructions:

Preheat oven to 425 and prepare baking dish

In a bowl mix together the olive oil, apple cider vinegar, and brown sugar; in another bowl pour in cornmeal. Dip the chicken in liquids and then in the cornmeal, cook 35-40 minutes at 425.

While not backed by science, numerous home remedies hold apple cider vinegar to help GERD. Although seemingly counter-intuitive vinegars are ok despite being acidic. This is not an endorsement or suggestion to use it as a cure or "quick-fix". There are various precautions one must take before it can be safely taken in lieu of medication, please seek out and confer with other sources before adding to your regimen

Recipe 3: Turkey and Tofu Green Beans

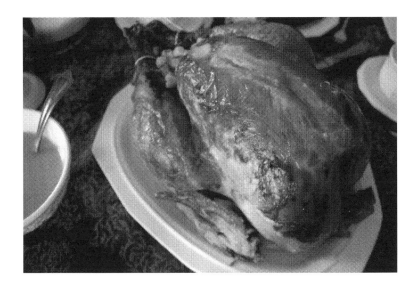

Also great with pork! Serves 3

List of Ingredients:

- 1 Tbsp. olive oil
- 4 turkey tenderloins
- ½ Tbsp. rosemary
- 3 cans, 14.5 oz., no salt added green beans
- 1 container firm tofu, cubed, drained, and dried
- 1/3 cup water
- 1 pinch cloves
- 1 Tbsp. honey
- ½ tsp. lemon juice

xxxxxxxxxxxxxxxxxxxxxxxxxxxxxxxxxxxx

Instructions:

In skillet over high heat cook the tenderloins and in the last few seconds sprinkle with rosemary. Meanwhile, brown tofu in pot, add beans, liquids, and seasonings and cook over high heat bringing it to a boil while stirring frequently. Reduce heat to low, cover, and simmer for 30-45 minutes.

Recipe 4: Burn Free Shrimp Pasta

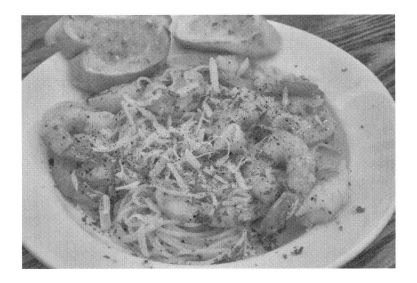

All of your friends and family will love this light and flavorful dish! 2 servings

List of Ingredients:

- 1 handful of linguine or angel hair pasta
- 1/3 - ½ pound medium shrimp, clean and tails removed
- ½ Tbsp. butter
- ½ Tbsp. olive oil
- 1/8 tsp. black pepper, onion powder, and garlic powder
- ½ Tbsp. diced rosemary
- Parmesan cheese (optional)

xxxxxxxxxxxxxxxxxxxxxxxxxxxxxxxxxxxx

Instructions:

Boil pasta noodles 8 minutes until "al dente", drain, and put aside for now. In skillet melt butter into olive oil and drop shrimp in, sprinkle with seasoning and cook 3-5 minutes or until no longer pink (overcooking will lead to a rubbery taste and texture).; remove, drain, and place on a paper towel covered plate. Let sit 3-4 minutes, mix into pasta, stir in diced rosemary, and sprinkle with cheese.

Recipe 5: White Lasagna

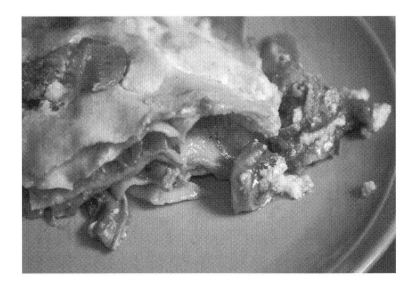

A tomato free classic dish! Makes 4-6 servings

List of Ingredients:

- 1 block cream cheese
- ½ stick butter
- ½ tsp. black pepper
- 1 /3 Tbsp. thyme and rosemary
- 1 pound lobster
- 2 cups spinach or corn (optional)
- 1 package parmesan cheese or feta cheese
- 1 package oven ready lasagna noodles

xxxxxxxxxxxxxxxxxxxxxxxxxxxxxxxxxx

Instructions:

Preheat oven to 350 and prepare a 9x9 casserole dish

In large pot melt together cream cheese and butter, mix in pepper, seasonings, lobster, and spinach/corn; in dish place a layer of noodles topped with a layer of sauce topped with a layer of cheese, and repeat until reaching top of dish. Cook 30 minutes at 350

Recipe 6: Thyme Ribs

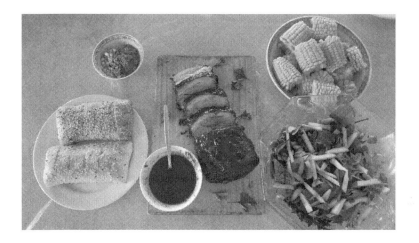

Excellent for grilling and outdoor gatherings! Makes 6 ribs

List of Ingredients:

- 6 beef ribs
- ½ cup of olive oil
- 1 Tbsp. brown sugar
- 1 Tbsp. thyme diced
- Black pepper

xxxxxxxxxxxxxxxxxxxxxxxxxxxxxxxxxxxxxxxx

Instructions:

Preheat oven to 350 and prepare baking tray

In a bowl or sauce pan mix oil, brown sugar, and thyme together; with a pastry brush paint onto ribs. Cook, uncovered, for 1 hour

Recipe 7: Piece O'Beef Kabobs

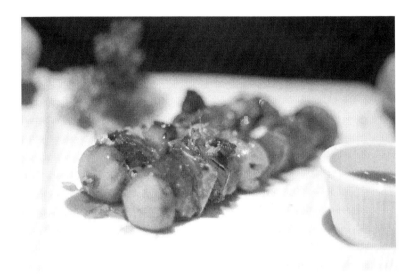

Remember to soak your skewers! Makes 8 kabobs or 4 servings

List of Ingredients:

- 4 cups worth of beef pieces
- 8 large tomatoes quartered **
- 4 large cucumbers cut into medium size rounds
- 2 large pineapple cut into large chucks
- Olive oil for drizzling

xxxxxxxxxxxxxxxxxxxxxxxxxxxxxxxxxxxxxxx

Instructions:

Preheat broiler and prepare broiling tray

In a skillet brown beef pieces and let sit on a paper towel at least 4-5 minutes. Fix skewers in the order listed above, drizzle with olive oil and put under the broiler 8-11 minutes turning once.

** Usually tomatoes are off limits but fresh are ok for most. However, if they do bother you consider mango, eggplant, or something similar.

Recipe 8: Honey Chicken

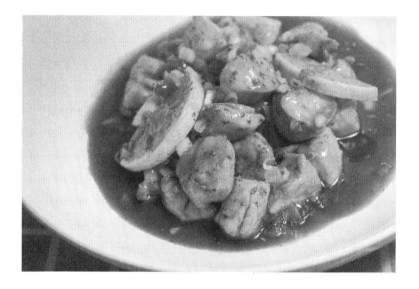

Works for white or dark meat! Makes 2 servings

List of Ingredients:

- 2 boneless, skinless chicken breasts
- 1 cup canned or thawed spinach
- 1/3 block cream cheese
- 2 Tbsp. olive oil
- 2/3 Tbsp. honey
- 1 Tbsp. apple cider vinegar
- ½ Tbsp. diced rosemary
- ½ tsp. orange peel (optional)
- ¼ - 1/3 tsp. Worchester sauce or vanilla extract

xxxxxxxxxxxxxxxxxxxxxxxxxxxxxxxxxxxx

Instructions:

Preheat oven to 350 and prepare baking tray

In plastic bags marinade the chicken breast overnight in olive oil, honey, a.c. vinegar, rosemary, orange peel, and Worchester sauce/vanilla extract. Squeeze as much water out of spinach as possible; in a bowl mix together spinach and cream cheese and set aside. Pound chicken and butterfly, spoon spinach mix inside and close chicken.

Bake, uncovered, 1 hour

Recipe 9: Spinach and Shrimp Parmesan Linguine

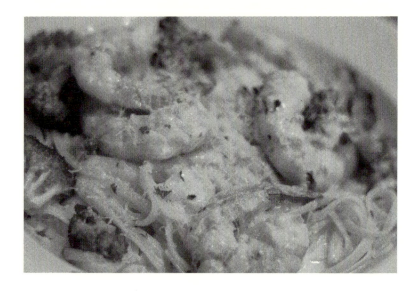

Excellent dish for serving guests; makes 4 servings

List of Ingredients:

- 3 cup shrimp, clean, deveined and tails removed
- 1/3 Tbsp. olive oil
- 1 dash red pepper flakes
- 2 cups spinach
- 1 ½ cup water
- 1/3 cup apple cider vinegar
- ¼ Tbsp. honey
- 1 dash cinnamon (optional)
- 6-8 oz. linguine
- Low fat Parmesan cheese

xxxxxxxxxxxxxxxxxxxxxxxxxxxxxxxxxxxxxxx

Instructions:

In skillet over the olive oil and red pepper flakes cook shrimp until no longer pink, approx. 2-4 minutes, and set aside on paper towel. In large pot place spinach, water, apple cider vinegar, cinnamon, and honey; bring to boil, reduce heat, and let simmer checking frequently and stirring. Meanwhile, boil linguine until al dente, drain but do not rinse. Add shrimp and linguine to spinach, stir well and serve

Recipe 10: GERD Stroganoff

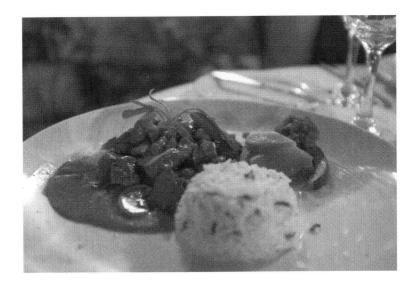

Avoid high fat, marbled cuts of beef; makes 4 servings

List of Ingredients:

- ½ Tbsp. olive oil
- 2 cups thin strips of steak
- ½ block of cream cheese cut into cubes
- 1 cup bok choy, kale, or spinach
- 1 small can mushroom, drained
- 1/6 tsp. cloves
- 2 ½ - 3 cups cooked wide egg noodles
- ¼ cup water, if needed**

xxxxxxxxxxxxxxxxxxxxxxxxxxxxxxxxxxxxxx

Instructions:

Fill crockpot with oil, steak strips, cream cheese, greens, mushrooms, and cloves. Cook on high 30 minutes, stir well, and continue cooking 30 more minutes. When there is ten minutes left for the crockpot cooking time, boil noodles 8 minutes, drain but do not rinse, pour into crockpot and mix well.

**This recipe does not require an abundance of liquid for you will end up with a soggy meal. However, if mix appears overly dry add water ¼ cup at a time.

Chapter IV - Stews

Recipe 1: Chickpea and Spinach Stew

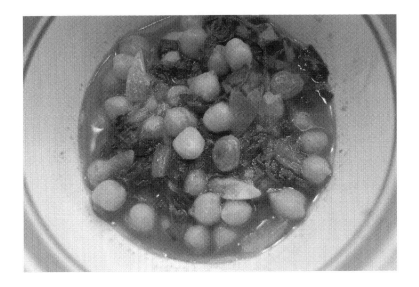

Try different types of beans such as cannellini and great northern; makes 9-11 servings

List of Ingredients:

- 2 cans low sodium chickpeas (garbanzo beans), washed and dried
- ½ Tbsp. olive oil
- 3 cups low sodium, low fat beef broth
- 1 cup spinach leaves
- 1 large sweet potato diced
- 1 tsp. black pepper

xxxxxxxxxxxxxxxxxxxxxxxxxxxxxxxxxxxx

Instructions:

Prepare crockpot

Place all ingredients and liquids into chamber and cook on high 1 hours.

Recipe 2: Pork and Sweet Potato Stew

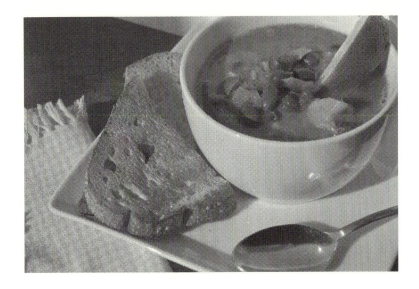

Great opportunity to add ingredients and spices that don't hurt! Makes 9-12 servings

List of Ingredients:

- 1-pound Fat free pork for stew pieces, or, 2-4 pork tenderloins cubed
- 2-3 sweet potatoes cubed, or seasonal foods like roasted butternut squash
- 4 cups beef broth
- 1 ½ Tbsp. all-purpose flour
- ½ Tbsp. diced oregano
- 1/3 Tbsp. diced thyme
- ½ Tbsp. parsley
- 1 dash blue monde spice (a mix of onion powder, garlic powder, and celery salt); only if you can handle it not necessary

xxxxxxxxxxxxxxxxxxxxxxxxxxxxxxxxxx

Instructions:

Prepare foods and crockpot, do not skip or skimp the draining it is very important to remove excess grease and oil. Your stomach will thank you!

Brown pork pieces and let drain on paper towel 4-5 minutes. Put all ingredients into chamber and cook on high 1 hour

Recipe 3: Beef and Broccoli Stew Version 2

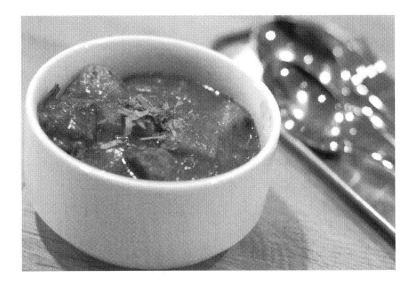

Try different types of rice for new dimensions of flavors!

Makes 9-11 servings

List of Ingredients:

- 1 ½ cups rice
- 1-pound beef strips
- 1 head of broccoli chopped
- 1/3 cup diced scallions
- Olive oil
- 1 tsp. celery salt
- ½ tsp. black pepper
- 4 cup low sodium, low fat cup beef broth

xxxxxxxxxxxxxxxxxxxxxxxxxxxxxxxxx

Instructions:

In a crockpot add olive oil, steak strips, cooked rice, broccoli, scallions, spices and seasonings, and broth. Cook on high 45 minutes to 1 hour.

Recipe 4: Beef and Broccoli Stew

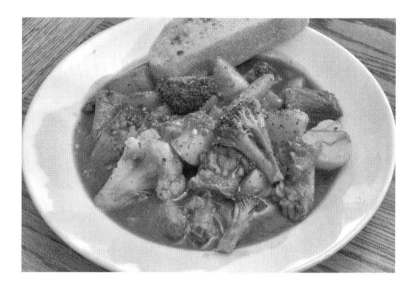

A low-fat, pain free twist on an old favorite! Makes 9-12 servings

List of Ingredients:

- 1-pound lean beef pieces for stew
- 1 can diced potatoes
- 1 head chopped broccoli
- ½ cup matchstick carrots
- 1 tsp. low fat soy sauce (can substitute with Worchester sauce if necessary)
- 4 cups low sodium beef broth
- 1 dash blue monde spice
- 1 Tbsp. all-purpose flour
- Prepare foods and crockpot, do not skip or skimp the draining it is very important to remove excess grease and oil. Your stomach will thank you!

xxxxxxxxxxxxxxxxxxxxxxxxxxxxxxxxxxx

Instructions:

Brown beef pieces and let drain on paper towel 4-5 minutes. Put all ingredients into chamber and cook on high 1 hour

Recipe 5: Cornmeal Veggie Stew

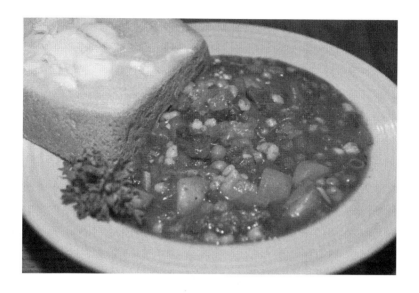

Always use low sodium stocks and broths! Makes 8-11 servings

List of Ingredients:

- 2 cans veggie mix
- 4 cups vegetable broth***
- ½ cup diced celery (if not included in the veg mix)
- 1 Tbsp. cornmeal
- ¼ tsp. black pepper

xxxxxxxxxxxxxxxxxxxxxxxxxxxxxxxxxxxx

Instructions:

Prepare foods and crockpot

Place all ingredients into chamber and cook on low 1-2 hours

***- chicken or beef broth can be substituted

Recipe 6: Chicken and Herbed Biscuits

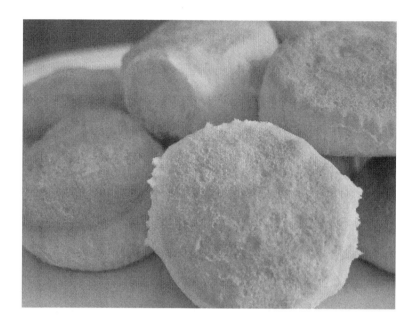

Great for busy nights! Makes 9-12 servings

List of Ingredients:

- 2 boneless, skinless chicken breast or thighs shredded
- 1 can condensed cream of chicken soup
- 4 cups low sodium chicken broth
- 1 stick butter
- 2 Tbsp. diced rosemary, parsley, basil, and oregano
- 1-2 cans frozen biscuits

xxxxxxxxxxxxxxxxxxxxxxxxxxxxxxxxx

Instructions:

To allow ample re-hardening time fix the butter a few hours before the chicken. In a pan melt the butter and add the spices, remove from heat and let sit 15-20 minutes pour into a freezer safe dish and freeze 2-4 hours or until hardened then place in refrigerator. In crockpot along with condensed soup and broth cook the chicken on high for 30-35 minutes, remove, shred, return and cook thirty more minutes.

Recipe 7: Herbed Chicken Stew

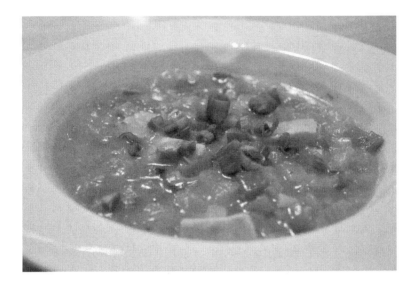

Better the second day! Makes 9-11 servings

List of Ingredients:

- ½ Tbsp. butter
- ¼ cup diced celery
- ¼ cup diced onion
- 1 cup shredded or cubed chicken breast or thigh
- 4 cups chicken broth
- 1 can condensed cream of chicken soup
- 1 can corn
- 2 cup bok choy, spinach, or kale
- ½ Tbsp. parsley, oregano and rosemary

xxxxxxxxxxxxxxxxxxxxxxxxxxxxxxxxxx

Instructions:

In crockpot melt butter and sauté onion and celery; add chicken, broth, cream of chicken soup, corn, and greens.

Cook on low 1-2 hours

Recipe 8: Bok Choy Stew

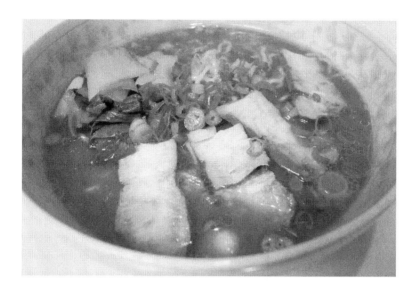

Many substitute options are available with this recipe, get creative! Makes 9-11 servings

List of Ingredients:

- Lean pork or beef pieces for stew
- 3-4 cups chopped bok choy, washed and dried
- 1 can corn
- 1 can black beans, washed and dried (optional)
- 2/3 cup diced mushrooms
- 4 cups beef broth
- 1 Tbsp. all-purpose flour
- Prepare foods and crockpot, do not skip or skimp the draining it is very important to remove excess grease and oil. Your stomach will thank you!

xxxxxxxxxxxxxxxxxxxxxxxxxxxxxxxxxx

Instructions:

Brown protein pieces and let drain on paper towel 4-5 minutes. Put all ingredients into chamber and cook on high 1 hour

Recipe 9: Shrimp and Corn Stew

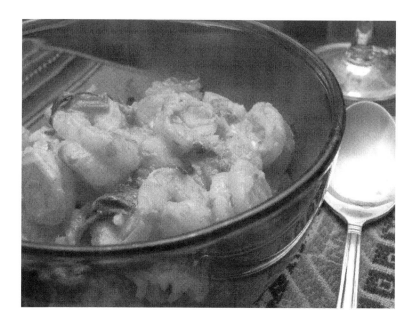

Fresh or frozen shrimp works! Makes 8-11 servings

List of Ingredients:

- ½ pound shrimp, cleaned, de-tailed, and diced
- 2 cans cream corn
- 6 oz. cream cheese
- 1 package crushed butter crackers
- 1 Tbsp. brown sugar
- 1 dash vanilla extract or Worchester sauce

xxxxxxxxxxxxxxxxxxxxxxxxxxxxxxxxx

Instructions:

Prepare foods and crockpot

Place all ingredients into chamber and cook on low 1-2 hours

Recipe 10: Ham and Broccoli Stew

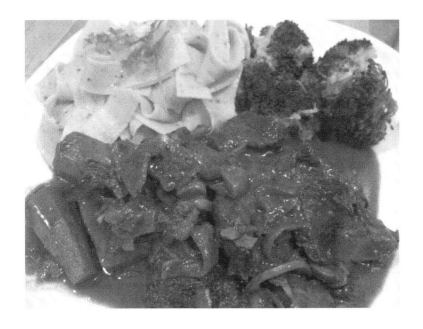

"Binge" worthy! Makes 8-11 servings

List of Ingredients:

- 1 cup diced ham
- ½ head of broccoli chopped
- ½ can diced potatoes
- 2 diced celery stalks or ½ Tbsp. celery salt
- 1 can condensed cream of mushroom soup
- 1 can condensed cream of broccoli soup
- 1 dash Worchester sauce
- 2 cups water
- 2 cups low sodium beef or chicken broth

XXXXXXXXXXXXXXXXXXXXXXXXXXXXXXXX

Instructions:

Prepare foods and crockpot

Place all ingredients into chamber and cook on low 1-2 hours

Chapter V - Snacks and Desserts

Recipe 1: GERD Approved Banana Bread

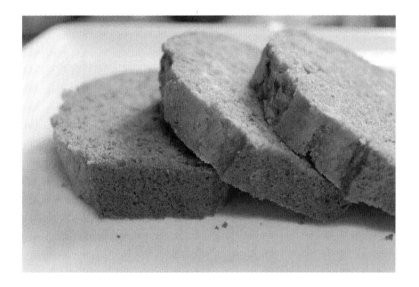

Makes a great gift! Makes 1 loaf, approx. 7-9 servings

List of Ingredients:

- 2 mashed bananas
- 2 egg whites
- 1 tsp. cinnamon
- 1/8 tsp. cloves
- 1 Tbsp. pecans pieces or walnuts
- 2 cups all-purpose flour
- 12 tsp. baking powder
- 1 tsp. baking soda
- 1/3 cup brown sugar
- 1 Tbsp. sugar
- 1 cup applesauce

xxxxxxxxxxxxxxxxxxxxxxxxxxxxxxxxxxxxx

Instructions:

Preheat oven to 350 and prepare bread tin

In one bowl mix dry ingredients and slowly beat in egg whites, applesauce, banana, and nuts; bake 45 minutes

Recipe 2: Chicken Pot Pie Muffins

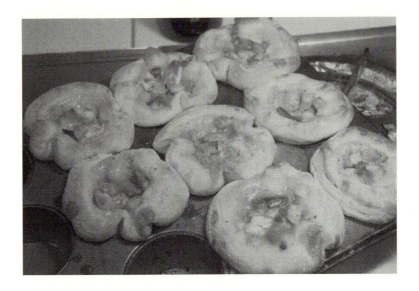

A creative way to use up leftovers! Makes 12-15

List of Ingredients:

- 1 package phylo dough
- 1 boneless, skinless chicken breast or thigh diced
- 1 can low sodium veggie mix
- 1 can low sodium condensed cream of chicken soup
- 1 tsp. celery salt
- 1 tsp. garlic and parsley seasoning

xxxxxxxxxxxxxxxxxxxxxxxxxxxxxxxxxxxx

Instructions:

Prepare muffin molds and preheat oven to 375

In a bowl mix together chicken, veggie mix, cream soup, and seasonings. Lay dough on flat surface and using the open end of a standard glass cup cut the dough into circles: place inside muffin holes. Fill each muffin with a large spoonful of mixture and cover with dough circle. Pierce top with fork to allow steam to escape and cook 18-22 minutes.

Recipe 3: Vanilla Ice Cream Strawberry Cake

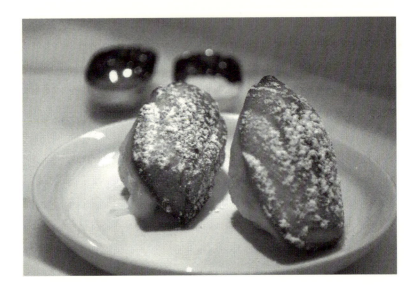

A great little dessert for all to enjoy! Makes 1 cake, approx. 4-5 servings

List of Ingredients:

- 1 Package vanilla cream wafers
- 1 tub low fat whip cream
- 1 tub fresh strawberries
- Strawberry syrup
- Strawberry ice cream

XXXXXXXXXXXXXXXXXXXXXXXXXXXXXXXXX

Instructions:

Place 7 vanilla cream wafers side by side, top with ice cream and syrup, repeat 4-5 more times. Frost with whipped topping, cover with foil and let sit in freezer 45-60 minutes; remove, put syrup on top and serve.

Recipe 4: Apple Crumble Muffins

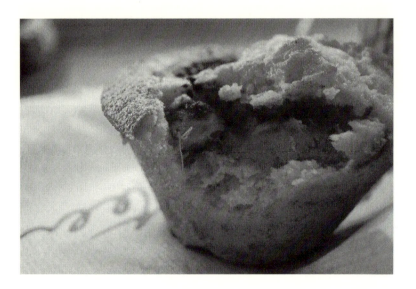

Great with coffee! Makes 12

List of Ingredients:

- 1 vanilla angel food cake mix
- 1 large can of apple pie filling
- Apple pie spice
- Brown sugar
- Graham cracker crumbs
- Ground pecans

xxxxxxxxxxxxxxxxxxxxxxxxxxxxxxxxxxxx

Instructions:

Mix cake mix and pour into muffin molds. In separate bowl, mix together apples, and spice; spoon on top of cake mix. In another bowl mix together brown sugar, graham cracker crumbs, and ground pecans; sprinkle on top of muffins. Bake 30-35 minutes

Recipe 5: Italian Half's

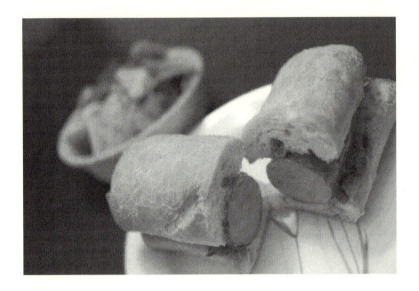

Kids of all ages love them! Makes 4 half's, or, 2 serving

List of Ingredients:

- 2 tsp. olive oil
- 2 Tbsp. skim milk ricotta cheese or parmesan cheese
- Italian seasoning
- 1 fresh large tomato ***
- 2 ciabatta roll cut in half

xxxxxxxxxxxxxxxxxxxxxxxxxxxxxxxxxxxx

Instructions:

Turn on broiler and prepare baking sheet

Separate roll and drizzle olive over half. Spread with ricotta cheese, sprinkle with seasoning, and tomato. Cook under broiler for 2-4 minutes

*** Fresh tomatoes are usually ok, but, if they cause flaring try eggplant instead

Recipe 6: Orange Bites

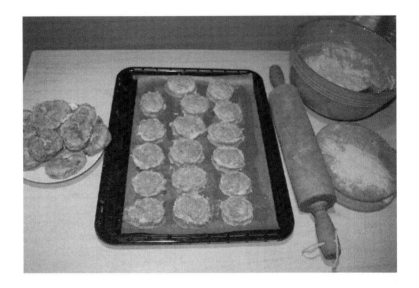

Great with ice cream! Makes 22-24

List of Ingredients:

- 1 vanilla cake mix, use apple sauce instead of oil
- ¼ cup brown sugar
- 1 Tbsp. honey
- 1 tsp. lemon juice
- 1 large can orange marmalade

xxxxxxxxxxxxxxxxxxxxxxxxxxxxxxxxxxxx

Instructions:

Prepare 11x8 casserole dish or silicon brownie molds and preheat oven to 350

In bowl mix together brown sugar, honey, lemon juice, and marmalade and refrigerate until ready use; in separate bowl, make cake mix according to package directions. Fill molds or dish with cake mix and spoon marmalade mixture on top; cook 30-35 minutes if using casserole dish, 20-25 minutes if using molds

Recipe 7: Baked Shrimp Won Tons

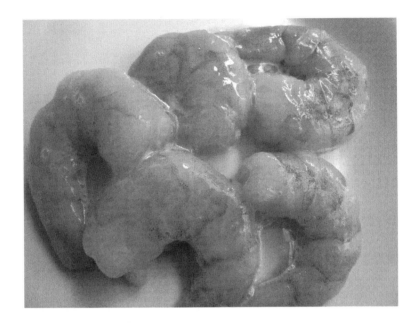

Try with a low-fat dipping sauce! Makes 8-10

List of Ingredients:

- ½ cup medium-large shrimp diced cleaned, deveined and de-tailed
- 1 cup broccoli slaw
- ½ cup diced water chestnuts
- 1 Tbsp. of grated or minced ginger
- ½ Tbsp. Worcester sauce

xxxxxxxxxxxxxxxxxxxxxxxxxxxxxxxxxxxxx

Instructions:

Preheat oven to 400 and prepare a baking sheet

Layout Won Ton wrappers, mix all ingredients in a large bowl, and spoon mixture into center, seal edges with water, and bake until golden in color.

Recipe 8: Baked Fritters

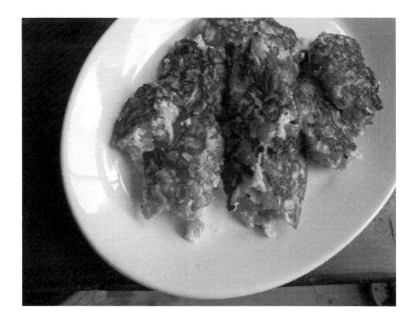

Even great without the seafood meat! Makes 15-17

List of Ingredients:

- ½ pound medium shrimp, cleaned, deveined, and de-tailed; lobster or clams
- 2 eggs
- 1 tsp. almond extract
- 1 cup all-purpose flour
- 2 tsp. tapioca starch
- 2 Tbsp. low fat milk
- 1/3 cup Italian breadcrumbs
- ½ Tbsp. Italian seasoning

xxxxxxxxxxxxxxxxxxxxxxxxxxxxxxxxxxx

Instructions:

Prepare baking tray and preheat oven to 425

Combine all ingredients, except for seafood, into a bowl and mix well. Dice seafood and fold into mixture, stir well. Spoon mounds onto tray and bake 20-25 minutes.

Recipe 9: Baked Vegetarian Spring Rolls

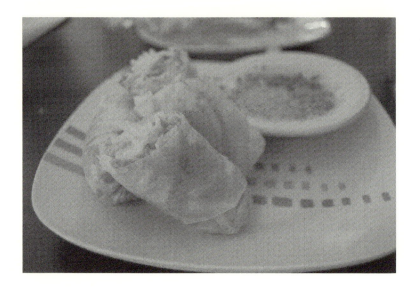

Excellent for a light snack between meals! Makes 10

List of Ingredients:

- 10 rice paper wrappers
- 1 carrot cut into chunks
- 1 cup cucumber cut into chunks
- 1 cup dice celery stalk cut into 3-inch pieces
- 1 cup cauliflower chunks
- 1/3 cup light olive oil
- 2 tsp. red wine vinegar
- 2 Tbsp. parsley, mint, and basil diced
- ½ tub low fat sour cream

xxxxxxxxxxxxxxxxxxxxxxxxxxxxxxxxxxxx

Instructions:

Preheat oven to 375 and prepare baking tray

In a bowl mix together sour cream and seasonings together, refrigerate when done. Place veggies into food processor and pulse 2-3 times 10-20 seconds on low. Pour in olive oil and red wine vinegar and stir; layout wrappers and spoon in the veggies. Cook 5-8 minutes and use sour cream mixture as a dip

Recipe 10: Black Cherry Yogurt Pops

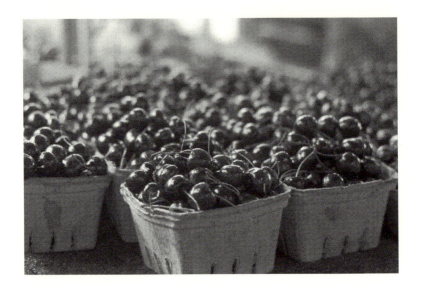

Great for hot days or an after-dinner treat! Makes 6-8

List of Ingredients:

- 2 ½ cup black cherry yogurt
- 1 cup cherry juice or Kool-Aid
- 1 package gelatin

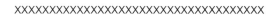

Instructions:

In a bowl mix yogurt, juice and gelatin; pour into molds and freeze 3-4 hours

Recipe 11: Tuna Salad Celery Dips

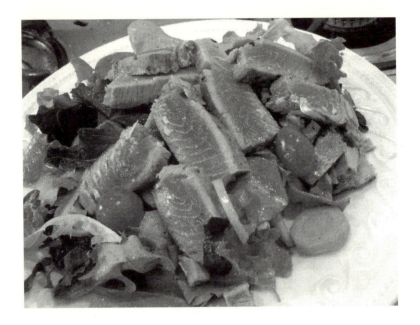

Try them with lobster, shrimp, ham, or chicken! Makes 8

List of Ingredients:

- 4 celery stalk each cut into 12 pieces
- 2 oz. cream cheese or ¼ cup low fat mayonnaise
- ½ Tbsp. diced basil, oregano, and mint
- 1 can tuna
- 1 tsp. oil or water

xxxxxxxxxxxxxxxxxxxxxxxxxxxxxxxxxxxxxxx

Instructions:

In a bowl mix together cream cheese, herbs, and tuna, spoon into celery centers. Make ahead by keeping in an air tight container in the refrigerator.

About the Author

Heston Brown is an accomplished chef and successful e-book author from Palo Alto California. After studying cooking at The New England Culinary Institute, Heston stopped briefly in Chicago where he was offered head chef at some of the city's most prestigious restaurants. Brown decide that he missed the rolling hills and sunny weather of California and moved back to his home state to open up his own catering company and give private cooking classes.

Heston lives in California with his beautiful wife of 18 years and his two daughters who also have aspirations to follow in their father's footsteps and pursue careers in the culinary arts. Brown is well known for his delicious fish and chicken dishes and teaches these recipes as well as many others to his students.

When Heston gave up his successful chef position in Chicago and moved back to California, a friend suggested he use the internet to share his recipes with the world and so he did! To date, Heston Brown has written over 1000 e-books that contain recipes, cooking tips, business strategies for catering companies and a self-help book he wrote from personal experience.

He claims his wife has been his inspiration throughout many of his endeavours and continues to be his partner in business as well as life. His greatest joy is having all three women in his life in the kitchen with him cooking their favourite meal while his favourite jazz music plays in the background.

Author's Afterthoughts

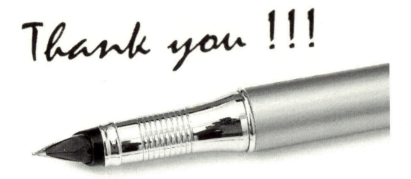

Thank you to all the readers who invested time and money into my book! I cherish every one of you and hope you took the same pleasure in reading it as I did in writing it.

Out of all of the books out there, you chose mine and for that I am truly grateful. It makes the effort worth it when I know my readers are enjoying my work from beginning to end.

Please take a few minutes to write an Amazon review so that others can benefit from your opinions and insight. Your review will help countless other readers make an informed choice

Thank you so much,

Heston Brown